Hospice Medication Handbook

Hospice Medication Handbook

A Caregiver's Guide to Comfort Medications

Peter M. Abraham, BSN, RN

Hospice Medication Handbook
A Caregiver's Guide to Comfort Medications
Copyright © 2024 Peter M. Abraham, BSN, RN

All rights reserved. No part of this book may be reproduced or transmitted in any manner whatsoever without written permission, except for brief quotations embodied in critical articles and reviews. This book is a work of nonfiction intended for educational purposes only.

This book is a work of non-fiction. The views expressed are solely those of the author and do not necessarily reflect the publisher's opinions, and the publisher disclaims any responsibility for them as a result.

Contact Info: author@2abraham.com

First Edition: August 2024

Dedication

This book is dedicated to my wife Laura, who has stood by and with me from the time of our wedding, which occurred when I was still working in information technology through the ins and outs of nursing school, including all my tears from being out of school for over thirty years, and throughout all the ups and downs of my nursing career.

Table of Contents

Introduction _____ 1

The Need for Comfort Medications _____ 3

    What Causes Pain and Suffering at the End of Life? _____ 3

    Common Causes of Pain _____ 3

    Sources of Suffering _____ 3

    Recognizing Signs of Pain and Suffering _____ 4

    The Role of Comfort Medications _____ 4

    Common Types of Comfort Medications _____ 5

    Working with the Hospice Team _____ 5

Understanding "As Needed" or PRN Medications _____ 6

    What Does "As Needed" or PRN Mean? _____ 6

    Communicating with Your Hospice Team _____ 6

    Tracking Medication Use _____ 7

    The Importance of Training _____ 8

    Final Thoughts _____ 8

Common Areas Comfort Medication Help _____ 9

    Pain and Discomfort _____ 9

    Shortness of Breath _____ 10

    Anxiety, Agitation, and Restlessness _____ 11

    Nausea and Vomiting _____ 12

Constipation 12

Terminal Secretions 13

Morphine Concentrate *14*

    What is Morphine Concentrate? 14

    Common Myths about Morphine Concentrate 14

    How Morphine Concentrate Works 14

    Understanding Half-Life 15

    Dosing in Hospice Care 15

    Benefits of Morphine Concentrate 15

    Side Effects and Management 16

    Strategies to Minimize Side Effects 16

    How to Administer Morphine Concentrate 16

    Alternatives for Morphine-Allergic Patients 17

Lorazepam Intensol *18*

    What is Lorazepam Intensol? 18

    Special Considerations 18

    Common Myths about Lorazepam Intensol 19

    How Lorazepam Intensol Works 19

    Understanding Half-Life 19

    Dosing in Hospice Care 20

    Benefits of Lorazepam Intensol 20

    Side Effects and Management 20

Strategies to Minimize Side Effects _____ 21

How to Administer Lorazepam Intensol _____ 21

Alternatives for Benzodiazepine-Allergic Patients _____ 21

Haloperidol Lactate _____ *22*

What is Haloperidol Lactate? _____ 22

Special Considerations _____ 22

Common Myths about Haloperidol Lactate _____ 23

How Haloperidol Lactate Works _____ 23

Understanding Half-Life _____ 23

Dosing in Hospice Care _____ 24

Benefits of Haloperidol Lactate _____ 24

Side Effects and Management _____ 24

Strategies to Minimize Side Effects _____ 25

How to Administer Haloperidol Lactate _____ 25

Alternatives for Haloperidol-Allergic Patients _____ 25

Anti-nausea (Anti-Emetic) Comfort Medications _____ *26*

Ondansetron (Zofran) _____ 26

How Ondansetron Works _____ 26

How to Take Ondansetron _____ 26

Prochlorperazine _____ 27

How Prochlorperazine Works _____ 27

Benefits and Side Effects of Prochlorperazine _____ 27

How to Take Prochlorperazine _____ 27

Additional Medications for Nausea _____ 28

Using Medications Together _____ 28

Tips for Caregivers _____ 28

Bisacodyl Suppository _____ 30

What is a Bisacodyl Suppository? _____ 30

How Bisacodyl Works _____ 30

Benefits and Side Effects _____ 30

How to Use a Bisacodyl Suppository _____ 30

Additional Strategies for Managing Constipation _____ 31

Tips for Caregivers _____ 31

Acetaminophen Suppository _____ 33

What Are Acetaminophen Suppositories? _____ 33

How They Work _____ 33

Benefits for Hospice Patients _____ 33

How to Use Acetaminophen Suppositories _____ 33

Dosage and Timing _____ 34

Other Ways to Provide Comfort _____ 34

When to Call for Help _____ 35

Common Medications for Terminal Secretions _____ 36

Understanding Terminal Secretions _____ 36

Medications Used to Manage Terminal Secretions _____ 36

Comparing the Medications _____ 39

Important Things to Remember _____ 39

Comfort Medication Management Best Practices _____ 40

Proper Storage of Comfort Medications _____ 40

Weekly Medication Review _____ 40

Keeping a Medication Administration Journal _____ 41

When to Give Specific Comfort Medications _____ 41

Final Thoughts _____ 42

Communication and Collaboration _____ 43

Working with Your Hospice Team _____ 43

Talking About Medication Changes with Family _____ 44

When to Reach Out for Help _____ 44

Final Thoughts _____ 45

Emotional Support for Caregivers: Taking Care of Yourself _ 47

Self-care Strategies: Nurturing Your Well-being _____ 47

Coping with Stress and Grief: Navigating Difficult Emotions _____ 48

Available Resources and Support Groups: You're Not Alone _____ 49

Creating Your Support Network: Building Your Circle of Care _____ 50

Final Thoughts _____ 50

Legal and Ethical Considerations in Hospice Care: Honoring Your Loved One's Wishes _____ 51

Understanding Advanced Directives: Planning for Future Care _____ 51

Power of Attorney Responsibilities: Advocating for Your Loved One _____ 52

Making Informed Decisions About Comfort Care: Focusing on Quality of Life _____ 53

Final Thoughts _____ 54

The Dying Process at the End of Life _____ 55

The Transitioning Phase _____ 55

The Actively Dying Phase _____ 56

The Last Hours _____ 57

Conclusion _____ 58

Resources _____ 60

Author Bio _____ 62

Introduction

Welcome, dear reader.

If you've picked up this book, you're likely facing one of life's most challenging journeys - caring for a loved one in hospice. This path can feel overwhelming and filled with questions, uncertainties, and emotions. But I want you to know that you're not alone. This book is here to be your supportive companion, guide, and source of comfort during this difficult time.

Caring for someone in hospice is an act of profound love and courage. It's a journey that can bring you closer to your loved one, even as you prepare to say goodbye. You might feel sadness, fear, and perhaps even moments of peace or gratitude. All of these feelings are normal and valid. Remember, there's no "right" way to feel or to navigate this experience.

In the following pages, we'll explore the world of comfort medications together. These medications play a crucial role in hospice care, helping to manage pain, ease breathing difficulties, reduce anxiety, and address other symptoms that might arise. Understanding these medications can help you feel more confident in your caregiving role and ensure your loved one remains comfortable.

We'll discuss these medications, how they work, and when they might be used. We'll also discuss potential side effects and how to manage them. Don't worry if some of this information initially seems overwhelming—your hospice team will always guide and answer your questions.

It's important to note that each hospice agency decides what medications are included in their "comfort kit" (sometimes called an "e-kit," "emergency kit," or "crisis kit"). This book covers the most common comfort medications, but the specific medicines in your kit may vary. Always ask your hospice team about the medications they've provided and why. If you think your loved one might benefit from a different medication, don't hesitate to discuss this with your hospice provider.

Beyond medications, we'll also explore other aspects of hospice care. We'll discuss how to communicate effectively with your hospice team, make critical care decisions, and care for yourself while caring for others. Remember, your well-being matters, too.

As you read this book, remember that every journey is unique, just as every life is unique. This guide isn't meant to give you all the answers but to provide knowledge, tools, and reassurance as you walk this path with your loved one.

There may be times when you feel overwhelmed or unsure. That's okay. Caring for someone at the end of life is one of the most challenging things we can do. But it's also one of the most meaningful. Your love, care, and presence are the most precious gifts you can offer. Your efforts matter, even on the most challenging days.

So take a deep breath. Remember that you're not alone on this journey. This book, your hospice team, and your support network are here to help you. Let's begin this journey together with compassion, understanding, and hope. You're doing important work, and your loved one is fortunate to have you by their side.

The Need for Comfort Medications

While dying itself isn't painful, the illnesses that lead to hospice care often involve pain and suffering. Understanding this can help you better support your loved one as a caregiver or family member.

What Causes Pain and Suffering at the End of Life?

Pain and suffering near the end of life can come from many sources. By understanding these causes, you can better support your loved one with compassion and care.

Common Causes of Pain

1. **Illness-Related Pain:** • Cancer: Especially when it spreads to bones or other areas • Chronic conditions: Such as long-lasting arthritis • Organ failure: Affecting the heart, lungs, or kidneys
2. **Treatment-Related Pain:** • Recent surgeries: Pain may linger, especially if healing is slow • Chemotherapy and radiation: Can cause pain and other side effects
3. **Other Physical Causes:** • Digestive problems: Such as constipation, nausea, and vomiting • Breathing difficulties: Shortness of breath can be very distressing • Skin irritation: Itching and dryness, mainly if bedridden • Extreme Fatigue: Can make discomfort feel worse

Sources of Suffering

1. **Emotional and Psychological Factors:** • Anxiety and stress: Worries about death or the future • Depression: Feelings of sadness can intensify physical symptoms • Fear: Of the unknown or pain
2. **Social and Environmental Factors:** • Isolation: Feeling alone can increase distress • Changes in routine: Disruptions in daily habits add to the discomfort

3. **Spiritual and Existential Factors:** • Existential distress: Worrying about the meaning of life and death • Spiritual pain: Struggles with faith or beliefs

Understanding Pain and Suffering

Type	Description	How You Can Help
Physical Pain	Discomfort in the body caused by illness or treatment	Ensure medications are given as prescribed, and use comfort measures like positioning
Emotional Suffering	Mental distress, anxiety, or depression	Provide emotional support, listen without judgment, consider counseling
Spiritual Distress	Questioning beliefs, searching for meaning	Offer spiritual support, connect with clergy if desired

Recognizing Signs of Pain and Suffering

It's essential to watch for signs that your loved one might be in pain or distress, especially if they have trouble communicating. Look out for:

- Facial expressions: Grimacing, frowning, or looking tense
- Body language: Rigidity, clenching fists, or pulling away when touched
- Sounds: Groaning, sighing, or calling out
- Changes in behavior: Becoming agitated, restless, or withdrawn

The Role of Comfort Medications

Comfort medications play a crucial role in managing pain and suffering at the end of life. They can:

1. Relieve physical pain
2. Ease breathing difficulties
3. Reduce anxiety and agitation
4. Help with nausea and vomiting

5. Improve overall quality of life

Common Types of Comfort Medications

Medication Type	Purpose	Examples
Pain Relievers	Manage various types of pain	Liquid Morphine
Anti-Anxiety Medications	Reduce anxiety and promote calmness	Lorazepam Intensol
Anti-Nausea Medications	Control nausea and vomiting	Ondansetron, Prochlorperazine

Working with the Hospice Team

Remember, you're not alone in this journey. The hospice team is there to support both you and your loved one. They can:

- Adjust medications as needed
- Provide education on proper medication use
- Offer additional comfort measures
- Support you emotionally throughout the process

Understanding the causes of pain and suffering, recognizing the signs, and working closely with the hospice team can help ensure your loved one receives the best care and comfort during this challenging time.

Understanding "As Needed" or PRN Medications

When discussing medications, you might hear the terms "as needed" or "PRN" when caring for a loved one in hospice. Let's explore what this means and how it affects your caregiving role.

What Does "As Needed" or PRN Mean?

- PRN stands for "pro re nata," Latin for "as the situation arises."
- These medications are taken only when symptoms occur, not on a fixed schedule
- Your hospice nurse may specify limits, like "every two hours" (sometimes written as Q2H)

Important Points to Remember:

1. Use these medications only when your loved one is experiencing discomfort
2. Follow any instructions given by your hospice nurse about when to use them
3. Always keep track of when and how much medication you give

Communicating with Your Hospice Team

Your hospice nurse will guide you on how to use PRN medications:

- They may ask you to call before giving any medication
- Or, they might allow you to use them as needed without calling first
- Either way, always record when you use these medications

Scenario	What to Do
The nurse asks you to call first	Contact hospice before giving any PRN medication
The nurse allows use as needed.	Give medication when symptoms arise, then inform hospice.
Unsure about instructions	Always ask your hospice nurse for clarification.

Tracking Medication Use

Keeping a record of medication use is crucial. Consider using a tool like the Daily Hospice Care Planner available at https://www.amazon.com/dp/B0DCGFPXLF to:

- Document when medications are given
- Track symptom changes
- Communicate effectively with your hospice team

Why Comfort Medications Are Provided Early

You might wonder why these medications are given to you at the start of hospice care. Here's why:

1. **Preparedness:** Having medications on hand allows for quick response to symptoms
2. **Accessibility:** Not all pharmacies are open 24/7
3. **Variability in needs:** Some patients may need frequent doses, while others may not need any
4. **Peace of mind:** Knowing you have what you need can reduce anxiety

Remember: Hospice nurses don't carry these medications, so having them at your location is essential.

The Importance of Training

While this information is helpful, it doesn't replace hands-on training from your hospice provider:

- Different nurses may provide varying levels of training
- Always ask questions if you're unsure about anything
- This guide can be a helpful reference, especially during late-night emergencies

Type of Training	What to Expect	Your Role
Hands-on demonstration	Nurse shows how to administer medications	Practice under supervision, ask questions
Verbal instructions	Nurse explains when and how to use medications	Take notes, ask for clarification if needed
Written materials	Nurse provides informational handouts	Review carefully, and keep it in an accessible place

Final Thoughts

Caring for a loved one in hospice can be challenging, but you're not alone. Remember:

- Your hospice team is there to support you
- Don't hesitate to ask questions or seek help
- Keeping good records helps ensure the best care for your loved one
- Having comfort medications on hand provides peace of mind

We hope this information helps you feel more prepared and confident in your caregiving role. Remember, your compassion and care make a world of difference to your loved one during this journey.

Common Areas Comfort Medication Help

As a caregiver, understanding how comfort medications work can help you provide better care for your loved one. Let's explore the different areas these medications can assist with.

Pain and Discomfort

Morphine: A Versatile Pain Reliever

Morphine is a powerful medication that helps with various types of pain during end-of-life care. Here's how it works for different pain types:

1. **Visceral Pain** • Originates from internal organs • Often feels like cramping or aching • Morphine calms these deep pain signals
2. **Somatic Pain** • Comes from bones or muscles • Usually sharp or throbbing • Morphine effectively reduces these sensations
3. **Neuropathic Pain** • Caused by nerve damage • Feels like burning or stabbing • Morphine can help when used with other treatments
4. **Breakthrough Pain** • Sudden flare-ups of pain • Liquid morphine works quickly to relieve these spikes

How Morphine Works:

- Attaches to opioid receptors in the brain and spinal cord
- Blocks pain signals from reaching the brain
- Liquid form is absorbed quickly, providing fast relief
- Dosage can be easily adjusted for personalized pain management

Shortness of Breath

Both morphine and Lorazepam Intensol can help manage breathing difficulties. Let's look at how each medication works:

Morphine for Breathing:

- Reduces the feeling of breathlessness
- Decreases anxiety related to breathing difficulties
- Slows breathing rate for more controlled breathing
- Widens blood vessels around the lungs (vasodilation)

Morphine's Impact on Breathing Mechanics:

Effect	Benefit
Longer exhalations	Improves lung function
Easier deep breaths	Enhances overall comfort
Better oxygen exchange	It makes breathing more manageable.
Less breathing distress	Reduces effort needed to breathe

Lorazepam Intensol for Shortness of Breath:

1. The calming effect reduces anxiety-related breathlessness
2. Muscle relaxation can make breathing easier
3. Helps slow rapid, shallow breathing

Important Note: Lorazepam can slow breathing, so it must be used carefully, especially with other medications that affect the nervous system.

Anxiety, Agitation, and Restlessness

Several medications can help manage these symptoms:

Lorazepam Intensol:

- Reduces anxiety quickly
- Calms agitation
- Promotes relaxation to reduce restlessness

Haloperidol Lactate:

- Manages severe agitation
- Helps settle restlessness
- Can reduce anxiety-related distress

Morphine Concentrate:

- Eases anxiety by relieving pain
- Reduces agitation by promoting calm
- Helps with restlessness through its calming effects

Using Medications Together:

Your hospice nurse may recommend the following:

- Using two or more medications simultaneously for severe symptoms
- Rotating medications throughout the day for consistent symptom control

Nausea and Vomiting

Several medications can help manage nausea and vomiting:

Medication	How It Works	Best For
Ondansetron	Blocks nausea-triggering chemicals	Nausea from chemo, radiation, surgery
Prochlorperazine	Blocks dopamine receptors	Various types of nausea
Haloperidol Lactate	Blocks dopamine receptors	Severe, treatment-resistant nausea
Lorazepam Intensol	Calms the brain and nerves	Anxiety-related nausea

Your hospice nurse may suggest using these medications together or in rotation for effective symptom management.

Constipation

Bisacodyl Suppositories:

- Stimulate intestinal muscles
- Increase fluid in intestines
- Usually work within 15 minutes to several hours

Additional Strategies:

- Drink warm prune juice
- Increase fiber intake
- Stay hydrated (4-6 glasses of water daily)

Your nurse may recommend combining medication with these strategies for better relief.

Terminal Secretions

Medications to manage terminal secretions (often called "death rattle"):

1. **Atropine** • Given as sublingual drops • Works quickly to reduce secretions
2. **Hyoscyamine** • Available in oral and sublingual forms • Can provide mild sedation
3. **Glycopyrronium** • Given orally • Less likely to cause confusion
4. **Scopolamine Patches** • Placed behind the ear • Provides continuous relief over several days

Non-Medication Approach:

- Reposition the patient to help secretions drain naturally

Remember, your hospice team is there to guide you through using these medications. Don't hesitate to ask questions or seek clarification when needed. Your care and attention make a significant difference in your loved one's comfort during this challenging time.

Morphine Concentrate

As a caregiver, understanding morphine concentrate can help you provide better care for your loved one. Let's explore this vital medication together.

What is Morphine Concentrate?

Morphine concentrate, also known as liquid morphine or Roxanol, is a powerful medication used in hospice care. It helps manage:

- Severe pain
- Shortness of breath
- Terminal agitation and restlessness

This medication changes how the brain and nervous system respond to pain, making it essential for keeping your loved one comfortable.

Common Myths about Morphine Concentrate

It's natural to have concerns about using morphine. Let's address some common myths:

Myth	Truth
Morphine accelerates death	Morphine relieves pain and discomfort, improving quality of life. It doesn't hasten death when used correctly.
Patients will become addicted.	In hospice care, the focus is on comfort. Physical dependence is not the same as addiction.
Morphine is only for cancer pain.	Morphine effectively manages various types of severe pain, not just cancer-related pain.

How Morphine Concentrate Works

1. **Binding to Receptors:** Morphine attaches to specific brain and spinal cord receptors.
2. **Pain Reduction:** This attachment reduces the perception of pain.

3. **Quick Action:** In liquid form, it works faster than pills, providing quicker relief.

Understanding Half-Life

The half-life of morphine is 2 hours. This means:

- After 2 hours, half of the medication is still working in the body
- After 4 hours, a quarter of the original dose is active
- This short half-life allows for flexible dosing to manage changing pain levels

Example: If your loved one receives 10 mg of liquid morphine at 8:00 AM:

- At 10:00 AM, 5 mg is still active
- At 12:00 PM, 2.5 mg is active
- At 2:00 PM, 1.25 mg is active

Dosing in Hospice Care

It's essential to understand the difference between toxic doses and common hospice doses:

- **Daily Maximum Toxic Dose:** Above 1,600 mg daily
- **Common Hospice Starting Doses:** 5 mg to 10 mg every 2 to 4 hours

Even 10 mg every hour (240 mg daily) is only 15% of the maximum daily dose. Your hospice team will carefully manage the dosage to ensure your loved one's comfort and safety.

Benefits of Morphine Concentrate

Morphine concentrate offers several benefits in hospice care:

1. **Pain Relief:** Provides significant comfort by managing severe pain

2. **Easier Breathing:** Helps ease respiratory distress, making breathing less difficult
3. **Calming Effect:** Reduces anxiety and agitation, promoting relaxation

Side Effects and Management

Like all medications, morphine can have side effects. Here are common ones and how to manage them:

Side Effect	Management Strategy
Constipation	Encourage fluids and fiber-rich foods, and use prescribed laxatives.
.Nausea and Vomiting	Use anti-nausea medications as prescribed.
Drowsiness	Monitor and report to the hospice team, may adjust dosing.
Dry Mouth	Offer ice chips, moisturize lips, and use oral swabs.
Confusion	Monitor and report to the hospice team, may adjust dosing.

Strategies to Minimize Side Effects

1. **Start Low, Go Slow:** Begin with a low dose and gradually increase as needed
2. **Stay Hydrated:** Encourage fluids when possible
3. **Monitor Closely:** Keep track of side effects and report to your hospice team
4. **Use Additional Medications:** As prescribed, to manage side effects

How to Administer Morphine Concentrate

Morphine concentrate can be given in two main ways:

1. **Buccal Administration:** • Place between the gum and cheek • Allows absorption through the mouth's lining • Often preferred due to less taste.

2. **Sublingual Administration:** • Place under the tongue • Absorbed quickly into the bloodstream • May have a stronger taste.

Alternatives for Morphine-Allergic Patients

If your loved one is allergic to morphine, other options are available:

- Hydromorphone: Similar to morphine but more potent
- Methadone: Long-acting, helpful for chronic pain
- Fentanyl: Available in patches for continuous pain relief

Remember, your hospice team is there to guide you through this process. They can answer questions, address concerns, and ensure your loved one receives the best care. Your dedication as a caregiver makes a difference in your loved one's comfort and quality of life during this journey.

Lorazepam Intensol

As a caregiver, understanding Lorazepam Intensol can help you better care for your loved one. Let's explore this vital medication together.

What is Lorazepam Intensol?

Lorazepam Intensol is a concentrated liquid form of lorazepam, a medication in the benzodiazepine class. It's beneficial in hospice care for managing:

- Anxiety
- Agitation
- Shortness of breath
- Nausea
- Seizures

This medication enhances the effects of a natural calming chemical in the brain, helping your loved one feel more relaxed and comfortable.

Special Considerations

Caution for Patients with Dementia or Parkinson's Disease: If your loved one has dementia or Parkinson's disease, Lorazepam Intensol should be used with extra care. It can sometimes:

- Increase confusion
- Raise the risk of falls
- Worsen symptoms of these conditions

Always consult with your hospice provider before starting this medication.

Common Myths about Lorazepam Intensol

Let's address some common misconceptions:

Myth	Truth
Lorazepam Intensol causes excessive sedation.	When used correctly, it manages symptoms without causing extreme drowsiness.
Patients will become addicted.	In hospice care, the focus is on comfort. Physical dependence is not the same as addiction.
Lorazepam Intensol is only for anxiety.	It effectively manages multiple symptoms, including agitation and nausea.

How Lorazepam Intensol Works

1. **Enhancing GABA:** Lorazepam boosts the effects of gamma-aminobutyric acid (GABA), a natural calming chemical in the brain.

2. **Promoting Relaxation:** This enhancement leads to calmness and relaxation.

3. **Quick Action:** In liquid form, it works faster than pills, providing quicker relief.

Understanding Half-Life

The half-life of Lorazepam Intensol is 8 to 12 hours. This means:

- After 8-12 hours, half of the medication is still working in the body
- This longer half-life allows for sustained symptom relief

Example: If your loved one receives 1 mg of Lorazepam Intensol at 8:00 AM:

- Between 4:00 PM and 8:00 PM, 0.5 mg is still active
- This helps maintain a consistent calming effect throughout the day

Dosing in Hospice Care

Understanding the difference between toxic doses and common hospice doses is essential:

- **Daily Maximum Toxic Dose:** Above 10 mg daily
- **Common Hospice Starting Doses:** 0.5 to 1.0 mg every 4 to 6 hours

Remember, even a dose of 1 mg every four hours (6 mg daily) is well below the maximum daily dose. Your hospice team will carefully manage the dosage to ensure your loved one's comfort and safety.

Benefits of Lorazepam Intensol

Lorazepam Intensol offers several benefits in hospice care:

1. **Anxiety Relief:** Provides quick and effective calming
2. **Easier Breathing:** Helps ease respiratory distress
3. **Calming Effect:** Reduces agitation and restlessness
4. **Nausea Control:** Can manage nausea when other medications aren't effective
5. **Seizure Management:** Helps control seizures for additional comfort and safety

Side Effects and Management

Like all medications, Lorazepam Intensol can have side effects. Here are common ones and how to manage them:

Side Effect	Management Strategy
Drowsiness	Monitor and report to the hospice team, may adjust dosing.
.Dizziness	Encourage hydration and assist with movement.
Weakness	Ensure a safe environment and assist with daily activities.
Unsteadiness	Use safety measures to prevent falls.
Confusion	Monitor and report to the hospice team, may adjust dosing.

Strategies to Minimize Side Effects

1. **Start Low, Go Slow:** Begin with a low dose and gradually increase as needed
2. **Monitor Closely:** Keep track of side effects and report to your hospice team
3. **Stay Hydrated:** Encourage fluids when possible
4. **Ensure Safety:** Create a safe environment to prevent falls and injuries

How to Administer Lorazepam Intensol

Lorazepam Intensol can be given in two main ways:

1. **Buccal Administration:** • Place between the gum and cheek • Allows for absorption through the mouth's lining
2. **Sublingual Administration:** • Place under the tongue • Absorbed quickly into the bloodstream

Alternatives for Benzodiazepine-Allergic Patients

If your loved one is allergic to benzodiazepines, other options are available:

- Hydroxyzine: An antihistamine that can help with anxiety and agitation
- Buspirone: An anti-anxiety medication that's not a benzodiazepine

Remember, your hospice team is there to guide you through this process. They can answer questions, address concerns, and ensure your loved one receives the best care. Your dedication as a caregiver makes a difference in your loved one's comfort and quality of life during this journey.

Haloperidol Lactate

Understanding Haloperidol Lactate can help you, as a caregiver, provide better care for your loved one. Let's explore this vital medication together.

What is Haloperidol Lactate?

Haloperidol Lactate is an antipsychotic medication commonly used in hospice care to manage:

- Agitation
- Delirium
- Severe nausea
- Anxiety

This medication works by balancing certain chemicals in the brain, helping to calm your loved one and improve their comfort.

Special Considerations

Caution for Patients with Lewy Body Dementia or Parkinson's Disease: If your loved one has Lewy Body Dementia or Parkinson's disease, Haloperidol Lactate should be used with extra care. It can sometimes:

- Worsen muscle rigidity
- Increase tremors
- Exacerbate other symptoms of these conditions

Always consult with your hospice provider before starting this medication.

Common Myths about Haloperidol Lactate

Let's address some common misconceptions:

Myth	Truth
Haloperidol Lactate is only for psychiatric patients.	While used in psychiatric care, it's also effective for managing symptoms in hospice patients.
It will make the patient a "zombie."	When used correctly, it manages symptoms without overly sedating the patient.
It's dangerous for elderly patients.	While caution is needed, it can be safely used under medical supervision to improve comfort.

How Haloperidol Lactate Works

1. **Blocking Receptors:** Haloperidol blocks specific receptors in the brain, particularly dopamine receptors.

2. **Reducing Agitation:** This blocking action helps reduce agitation and calm the patient.

3. **Controlling Nausea:** It also helps control severe nausea by affecting certain brain areas.

Understanding Half-Life

The half-life of Haloperidol Lactate is about 14 to 26 hours. This means:

- After 14-26 hours, half of the medication is still working in the body
- This longer half-life allows for sustained symptom relief

Example: If your loved one receives 1 mg of Haloperidol Lactate at 8:00 AM:

- Between 10:00 PM and 10:00 AM the next day, 0.5 mg is still active
- This helps maintain a consistent calming effect for an extended period

Dosing in Hospice Care

Understanding the difference between toxic doses and common hospice doses is essential:

- **Daily Maximum Toxic Dose:** Above 30 mg daily
- **Common Hospice Starting Doses:** 0.5 to 2.0 mg every 4 to 6 hours

Remember, even a dose of 2 mg every four hours (12 mg daily) is well below the maximum daily dose. Your hospice team will carefully manage the dosage to ensure your loved one's comfort and safety.

Benefits of Haloperidol Lactate

Haloperidol Lactate offers several benefits in hospice care:

1. **Anxiety Relief:** Provides quick and effective calming
2. **Agitation and Delirium Management:** Reduces restlessness and confusion
3. **Nausea Control:** Effective in managing severe nausea when other medications aren't working

Side Effects and Management

Like all medications, Haloperidol Lactate can have side effects. Here are common ones and how to manage them:

Side Effect	Management Strategy
Drowsiness	Monitor and report to the hospice team, may adjust dosing.
Dizziness	Encourage hydration and assist with movement.
Dry Mouth	Offer ice chips, moisturize lips, and use oral swabs.
Muscle Rigidity	Report to the hospice team; dose adjustment may be needed.
Tremors	Monitor and report to the hospice team, may adjust dosing.

Strategies to Minimize Side Effects

1. **Start Low, Go Slow:** Begin with a low dose and gradually increase as needed
2. **Monitor Closely:** Keep track of side effects and report to your hospice team
3. **Stay Hydrated:** Encourage fluids when possible
4. **Ensure Safety:** Create a safe environment to prevent falls and injuries

How to Administer Haloperidol Lactate

Haloperidol Lactate can be given in two main ways:

1. **Buccal Administration:** • Place between the gum and cheek • Allows for absorption through the mouth's lining
2. **Sublingual Administration:** • Place under the tongue • Absorbed quickly into the bloodstream

Alternatives for Haloperidol-Allergic Patients

If your loved one is allergic to Haloperidol, other options are available:

- Quetiapine (Seroquel): Less likely to cause muscle rigidity
- Olanzapine (Zyprexa): Effective for multiple symptoms with a lower risk of movement disorders
- Risperidone (Risperdal): Requires lower doses, making it easier to manage

Remember, your hospice team is there to guide you through this process. They can answer questions, address concerns, and ensure your loved one receives the best care. Your dedication as a caregiver makes a difference in your loved one's comfort and quality of life during this journey.

Anti-nausea (Anti-Emetic) Comfort Medications

Understanding anti-nausea medications can help you, as a caregiver, better comfort your loved one. Let's explore these essential medications together.

Ondansetron (Zofran)

What is Ondansetron?

Ondansetron is a powerful medication used to prevent nausea and vomiting. It benefits hospice patients who may experience these symptoms due to their condition or other medications.

How Ondansetron Works

1. **Blocking Serotonin:** Ondansetron stops a natural serotonin chemical from causing nausea.
2. **Quick Action:** It works in the brain and stomach to stop nausea signals.
3. **Fast Relief:** Most people feel the effects within 1.5 hours.

Benefits and Side Effects of Ondansetron

Benefits	Side Effects
Effectively reduces nausea and vomiting.	Headache
It helps patients feel more comfortable.	Dizziness
Available in easy-to-take forms	Constipation

Note: In rare cases, Ondansetron can affect heart rhythm. If your loved one has a heart condition, make sure to inform the hospice team.

How to Take Ondansetron

- **Forms:** Tablets, dissolvable tablets, or oral solutions

- **Dosage:** Your hospice team will determine the right amount for your loved one
- **Timing:** Often given as needed to control nausea

Prochlorperazine

What is Prochlorperazine?

Prochlorperazine is another medication that helps control nausea and vomiting, especially when other treatments aren't working well.

How Prochlorperazine Works

- It blocks dopamine receptors in the brain
- This action helps control nausea and vomiting signals

Benefits and Side Effects of Prochlorperazine

Benefits	Side Effects
Manages severe nausea and vomiting	Drowsiness
Provides relief when other medications don't work	Dizziness
	Dry mouth
	Muscle stiffness (at higher doses)

How to Take Prochlorperazine

- **Forms:** Oral tablets or suppositories
- **Dosage:** Given as needed, adjusted based on how your loved one responds
- **Timing:** Your hospice team will guide you on when to use it

Additional Medications for Nausea

Sometimes, your hospice team might suggest using other medications alongside Ondansetron or Prochlorperazine to enhance their effectiveness.

1. Lorazepam Intensol • Helps reduce anxiety-related nausea • Provides a calming effect • Can make other anti-nausea medications work better

2. Haloperidol Lactate • Used for severe nausea that doesn't respond to other treatments • Works similarly to Prochlorperazine

Using Medications Together

Your hospice nurse might suggest using these medications in different ways:

1. **Combined Use:** Sometimes, using more than one medication at a time can help control severe symptoms quickly.

2. **Rotation:** Different medications might be given at various times throughout the day to keep nausea under control.

Tips for Caregivers

1. **Keep a symptom diary:** Note when nausea occurs and which medications seem to help most.

2. **Offer small, frequent meals:** This can be easier on the stomach than large meals.

3. **Encourage hydration:** Small sips of water or ice chips can help prevent dehydration.

4. **Create a calm environment:** Reduce strong smells and provide a quiet, comfortable space.

5. **Communicate with your hospice team:** Let them know how the medications work and your concerns.

Remember, your role as a caregiver is invaluable. By understanding these medications and working closely with your hospice team, you're helping to ensure your loved one's comfort. Don't hesitate to ask questions or seek support when you need it. Your dedication makes a difference in your loved one's quality of life during this journey.

Bisacodyl Suppository

As a caregiver, you know that constipation can be uncomfortable and distressing for your loved one in hospice care. Bisacodyl suppositories offer a gentle and effective way to manage this issue, helping to improve comfort and quality of life. Let's explore this medication together.

What is a Bisacodyl Suppository?

Bisacodyl is a stimulant laxative used to treat occasional constipation. It comes in the form of a suppository, which is inserted rectally.

How Bisacodyl Works

1. **Stimulates intestinal muscles:** Helps move stool through the bowel
2. **Increases fluids in the intestines:** Softens the stool, making it easier to pass
3. **Quick action:** Usually results in a bowel movement within 15 to 60 minutes

Benefits and Side Effects

Benefits	Side Effects
Quick relief from constipation	Mild abdominal cramps
Prevents complications like fecal impaction	Rectal burning
Easy to use	Faintness (rare)

Note: Overuse can lead to dependency, where the body relies on the laxative for regular bowel movements. Always follow your hospice team's guidance on usage.

How to Use a Bisacodyl Suppository

Follow these steps to administer the suppository correctly:

1. Wash your hands thoroughly

2. Remove the suppository from its foil wrapper
3. Wet the tip with cold water for easier insertion
4. Have your loved one lie on their side with knees drawn up to the chest
5. Gently insert the suppository, pointed end first, into the rectum
6. Try to keep it in place for 15 to 20 minutes or until there's an urge to have a bowel movement
7. rewash your hands after administration

Dosage for Adults: Use one suppository once daily as needed or as directed by your hospice team.

Additional Strategies for Managing Constipation

While Bisacodyl suppositories can be very effective, your hospice nurse may also recommend other strategies to help manage constipation:

1. **Warm Prune Juice** • Contains natural laxatives • Can stimulate bowel movements • Offer 4-8 ounces, warmed for better taste and effect
2. **Increase Fiber Intake** • Add fruits, vegetables, and whole grains to the diet if possible • Helps add bulk to the stool • Makes passing stool easier
3. **Stay Hydrated** • Encourage drinking fluids, especially water • Helps keep stool soft • Aim for 6-8 glasses of fluid per day, if appropriate for your loved one's condition

Tips for Caregivers

- **Be gentle and patient:** Constipation can be uncomfortable and embarrassing for your loved one. Your understanding makes a big difference.
- **Maintain privacy:** Ensure your loved one has as much privacy as possible during bowel movements.

- **Keep a log:** Note bowel movements and any discomfort. This information can be helpful for your hospice team. The Daily Hospice Care Planner at https://www.amazon.com/dp/B0DCGFPXLF has a template for tracking bowel movements.

- **Watch for signs of constipation:** These may include decreased appetite, nausea, or abdominal discomfort.

- **Communicate with your hospice team:** Let them know how the suppositories work and any concerns you have.

Remember, your role as a caregiver is invaluable. By understanding how to use Bisacodyl suppositories and implementing additional strategies, you're helping to ensure your loved one's comfort. Don't hesitate to ask questions or seek support when you need it. Your dedication makes a difference in your loved one's quality of life during this journey.

Acetaminophen Suppository

When someone you care about is nearing the end of life, keeping them comfortable is essential. Fever and pain can cause distress, but there are gentle ways to help. One option is acetaminophen suppositories. Let's talk about how these can help your loved one feel better.

What Are Acetaminophen Suppositories?

Acetaminophen suppositories are medicines that are inserted into the rectum instead of swallowed. They contain the same active ingredient as Tylenol but in a form that melts at body temperature. This allows the medicine to be absorbed into the bloodstream through the rectal lining.

How They Work

- **Pain Relief**: Acetaminophen reduces pain signals in the brain
- **Fever Reduction**: It also helps lower body temperature when there's a fever
- **Gentle Action**: Works without irritating the stomach

Benefits for Hospice Patients

For people nearing the end of life, these suppositories can be helpful:

- **Easy to Use**: No need to swallow pills, which can be challenging for some patients
- **Reliable Relief**: Helps with mild to moderate pain and fever
- **Few Side Effects**: Generally very safe when used as directed

How to Use Acetaminophen Suppositories

Giving a suppository might initially feel strange, but it's not complicated. Here's a step-by-step guide:

1. Wash your hands thoroughly

2. Remove the suppository from its wrapper
3. If it feels hard, you can soften it by holding it in your hand for a minute
4. Help your loved one lie on their side with their top leg bent towards their stomach
5. Gently insert the suppository, rounded end first, about 1 inch into the rectum
6. Hold the buttocks together for a moment to keep the suppository in place
7. Encourage your loved one to stay lying down for about 15 minutes if possible
8. Wash your hands again

Dosage and Timing

Always follow the instructions given by your hospice nurse or doctor. Generally:

- Use one suppository every 4 to 6 hours as needed
- Don't use more than 4 in 24 hours unless directed by a healthcare provider

Other Ways to Provide Comfort

While acetaminophen suppositories can help, there are other things you can do to keep your loved one comfortable:

- Keep the room at a comfortable temperature
- Use light, breathable bedding
- Offer small sips of water or ice chips if they're able to swallow safely
- Gently apply a cool, damp cloth to the forehead if they have a fever
- Speak softly and reassuringly

When to Call for Help

If your loved one's pain or fever doesn't improve, or if you notice any unusual symptoms, don't hesitate to contact your hospice team. They're there to support you and ensure your loved one's comfort.

Remember, your care and presence are the most crucial comforts you can provide. Medical tools, like acetaminophen suppositories, support the loving care you're already giving.

Common Medications for Terminal Secretions

When a loved one is in their final days, you may notice a gurgling or rattling sound when they breathe. This is often called the "death rattle," though medical professionals refer to it as terminal secretions. While it can be upsetting to hear, it's essential to know that it usually doesn't bother your loved one. However, some medications can help reduce these secretions and make everyone more comfortable.

Understanding Terminal Secretions

Terminal secretions happen when someone can't clear fluids from their throat or lungs. This is common as the body's systems start to slow down. The sound you hear is air passing through these fluids.

Key points to remember:

- This is a normal part of the dying process
- It doesn't usually cause discomfort to your loved one
- Medications can help reduce secretions

Medications Used to Manage Terminal Secretions

Several medications can help reduce secretions. They all work in similar ways, but each has its characteristics. Let's look at four common options:

1. Atropine Drops

How it works: Atropine reduces the production of saliva and mucus.

Benefits:

- Acts quickly
- Easy to give (placed under the tongue)

Possible side effects:

- Dry mouth
- Blurred vision
- Faster heart rate

How it's given:

- Usually 1-2 drops under the tongue every 6 hours

2. Hyoscyamine (Levsin)

How it works: Hyoscyamine reduces secretions and can provide mild calming effects.

Benefits:

- Effective at reducing secretions
- May help your loved one feel calmer

Possible side effects:

- Dry mouth
- Dizziness
- Difficulty urinating

How it's given:

- Can be given under the tongue or as an injection under the skin
- Typical dose is 0.125 to 0.5 mg every 4 hours

3. Glycopyrronium (Robinul)

How it works: Glycopyrronium reduces secretions but doesn't cross into the brain as much as other options.

Benefits:

- Effective at reducing secretions
- Less likely to cause drowsiness

Possible side effects:

- Dry mouth
- Constipation

How it's given:

- Can be given by mouth or as an injection under the skin
- Typical dose is 1 mg by mouth or 0.2 to 0.4 mg under the skin every 4 hours

4. Scopolamine Patches

How it works: Scopolamine is delivered through a patch on the skin, providing continuous medication to reduce secretions.

Benefits:

- Provides long-lasting relief
- Easy to use (apply the patch)

Possible side effects:

- Dry mouth
- Drowsiness
- Blurred vision

How it's given:

- 1 or 2 patches applied to the skin
- Each patch lasts for 72 hours (3 days)

Comparing the Medications

To help you understand the differences between these medications, here's a comparison table:

Medication	How It's Given	How Often	Main Benefit	Main Side Effect
Atropine	Drops under tongue	Every 6 hours	Quick acting	Dry mouth
Hyoscyamine	Under tongue or injection	Every 4 hours	It may help with calming	Dizziness
Glycopyrronium	By mouth or injection	Every 4 hours	Less drowsiness	Constipation
Scopolamine	Skin patch	Every 72 hours	Long-lasting	Drowsiness

Important Things to Remember

1. **These medications are not usually started until secretions become noticeable.**

2. **Always follow the instructions given by your hospice team.** They will decide which medication is best and how much to use.

3. **Don't hesitate to ask questions.** Your hospice team is there to support you and your loved one.

4. **Other comfort measures can help, too.** Gently turning your loved one's head to the side or slightly elevating the head of the bed can sometimes help secretions drain naturally.

5. **Your presence is the most essential comfort.** While these medications can help manage symptoms, loving care matters most.

Remember, it's okay to feel overwhelmed or unsure. Caring for a loved one at the end of life is a profound and challenging experience. Your hospice team is there to support you every step of the way.

Comfort Medication Management Best Practices

When someone you love is in hospice care, managing their medications becomes an integral part of ensuring their comfort. It might initially feel overwhelming, but with some guidance and practice, you can help your loved one feel as comfortable as possible. Review some best practices to help you manage comfort medications effectively and confidently.

Proper Storage of Comfort Medications

Storing medications correctly is crucial for keeping them safe and effective. Here are some key points to remember:

1. **Find a cool, dry place**: Medications don't like heat or moisture. A drawer or cabinet away from windows and heat sources is often perfect.
2. **Keep them secure**: Make sure medications are out of reach of children and pets. A high shelf or a lockbox can be good options.
3. **Leave them in original packaging**: This helps avoid mix-ups and keeps critical information handy.
4. **Organize for easy access**: You might want to use a pill organizer or create a system that works for you and your loved one.

Remember, proper storage isn't just about following rules – it's about keeping your loved one safe and ensuring their medications work as intended.

Weekly Medication Review

Reviewing medications each week can help you stay on top of your loved one's changing needs. Here's a simple checklist you can follow:

- Check expiration dates on all medications
- Dispose of any expired medications safely
- Make sure current medications match the care plan

- Note any medications that are running low
- Write down any questions or concerns to discuss with the hospice nurse

This weekly check-in is an excellent opportunity to reflect on how the medications work and if any adjustments are needed. The Daily Hospice Care Planner includes a template for tracking refill needs.

Keeping a Medication Administration Journal

Keeping track of when medications are given and how they work is incredibly helpful. It allows you to share accurate information with the hospice team and helps ensure your loved one's comfort. Here's what to include in your journal:

What to Record	Why It's Important
Date and Time	Helps track medication schedule
Who Gave the Medication	Useful for coordinating care
Medication Name and Dose	Ensures correct medication is given
Reason for Giving	Helps track symptoms
How It Worked	Helps assess effectiveness

For the "How It Worked" part, note how your loved one seemed to feel at 30 minutes, 60 minutes, 90 minutes, and 2 hours after getting the medication. This information is precious for the hospice team. The Daily Hospice Care Planner has a template for tracking when medications are given and can be an excellent tool to ensure everyone is on the same page.

When to Give Specific Comfort Medications

Knowing when to give certain medications can help you respond quickly to your loved one's needs. Here are some general guidelines:

- **Pain Medications**: Give these when your loved one shows pain or discomfort, such as grimacing, moaning, or becoming restless.
- **Anti-Nausea Medications**: Use these if your loved one feels sick or is vomiting.
- **Anxiety Medications**: These can help if your loved one seems worried, agitated, or can't relax.

- **Medications for Secretions**: If you notice gurgling sounds when your loved one breathes, medications like atropine or scopolamine can help.

Always follow the specific instructions given by your hospice team. They know your loved one's unique situation and can guide you on the best medication timing.

Final Thoughts

Managing medications might feel like a big responsibility, but remember – you're not alone. Your hospice team is there to support you every step of the way. Don't hesitate to ask questions or share your concerns.

Your loving care and proper medication management can make a difference in keeping your loved one comfortable. Remember to take care of yourself, too, during this challenging time. Your well-being is just as important.

Communication and Collaboration

When someone you care about receives hospice care, communication becomes more critical than ever. It helps ensure your loved one gets the best possible comfort and support. Let's explore how you can work well with your hospice team, discuss medication changes, and know when to ask for help.

Working with Your Hospice Team

Your hospice team is like a group of helping hands, all reaching out to support you and your loved one. Here's how you can work together effectively:

1. **Get to know your team**: Take a moment to learn who's who. Your team might include:
    - Nurses
    - Doctors
    - Social workers
    - Chaplains
    - Home health aides
    - Volunteers

2. **Keep the lines open**: Don't be shy about asking questions or sharing worries. Your team wants to hear from you.

3. **Be honest about what's happening**: The more your team knows about your loved one's feelings, the better they can help.

4. **Follow the care plan**: Work with your team to create a proper plan, then do your best to follow it.

5. **Use what's offered**: Many hospice teams provide helpful resources like educational materials or support groups. These can be valuable, so take advantage of them.

Remember, you're not alone on this journey. Your hospice team is there to support you every step of the way.

Talking About Medication Changes with Family

When medications change, it's essential to keep everyone in the loop. Here are some tips for having these conversations:

- **Find the right moment**: Choose a quiet time when everyone can focus on the conversation.

- **Be open and honest**: Explain why the medication changes and what it might mean for your loved one.

- **Keep it simple**: Try to avoid medical jargon. If you need to use complex terms, explain what they mean.

- **Welcome questions**: Ensure everyone understands and feels comfortable asking for more information.

- **Listen to concerns**: Some family members might worry about changes. If necessary, listen to their concerns and seek answers from the hospice team.

- **Write it down**: Record medication changes to share with family members who couldn't attend the discussion.

The [Daily Hospice Care Planner: Organize, Communicate, and Provide Consistent Care](#) was developed with families in mind; consider this as an additional tool you can use to ensure the best care for your loved one.

When to Reach Out for Help

Your hospice team will visit regularly, but there may be times when you need help right away. Here are some situations when you should call your hospice team:

1. **New or worsening symptoms**: If your loved one experiences:
    - Increased pain
    - Trouble breathing
    - Severe nausea or vomiting
    - Sudden confusion or agitation

2. **Medication issues**: Call if:
    - A medication doesn't seem to be working
    - There are unexpected side effects
    - You're unsure about how to give a medication
    - You're running low on essential medications
3. **Falls or injuries**: Always report falls or injuries, even if they seem minor.
4. **Emotional distress**: Don't hesitate to contact someone if you or your loved one is struggling emotionally.
5. **Equipment problems**: Contact the hospice team if medical equipment isn't working right.
6. **End-of-life signs**: If you notice signs that might indicate the final stages of life, such as:
    - Decreased consciousness
    - Changes in breathing patterns
    - Decreased urine output
    - Skin color changes

Remember, there's no such thing as a "silly" question or concern. Your hospice team is available 24/7 and would much rather you call with a question than worry alone.

Final Thoughts

Good communication is like a bridge that connects you, your loved one, your family, and your hospice team. By strengthening this bridge, you can all work together to provide your loved one the best possible care and comfort.

It's okay to feel overwhelmed sometimes. Caring for someone in hospice can be challenging. But remember, you're not alone. Your hospice team is there to support you, answer your questions, and help you navigate this journey.

Your love, care, and attention to good communication can make a difference in your loved one's comfort and peace of mind. And that's a beautiful gift to give.

Emotional Support for Caregivers: Taking Care of Yourself

Caring for a loved one in hospice is a journey of love, but it can also be emotionally and physically challenging. It's important to remember that your well-being matters too. Let's explore ways to care for yourself while providing necessary care for your loved one.

Self-care Strategies: Nurturing Your Well-being

Taking care of yourself isn't selfish—it's necessary. Here are some strategies to help you stay healthy and balanced:

1. **Prioritize rest**
    - Aim for 7-9 hours of sleep each night
    - Take short naps when possible
    - Try relaxation techniques like deep breathing or meditation

2. **Maintain a healthy diet**
    - Eat regular, balanced meals
    - Stay hydrated
    - Limit caffeine and alcohol

3. **Move your body**
    - Take short walks to boost your mood and energy
    - Try gentle yoga or stretching
    - Consider chair exercises if you can't leave your loved one

4. **Take breaks**
    - Step outside for fresh air
    - Read a book or listen to music
    - Call a friend for a quick chat

5. **Practice mindfulness**
    - Focus on the present moment
    - Acknowledge your feelings without judgment
    - Try guided meditation apps or videos

Remember, taking care of yourself allows you to provide better care for your loved one. It's like putting on your oxygen mask first on an airplane—you need to be okay to help others.

Coping with Stress and Grief: Navigating Difficult Emotions

Caring for someone in hospice can bring up intense emotions. Here are some ways to cope:

- **Acknowledge your feelings**: It's normal to feel a range of emotions, including sadness, anger, guilt, or even relief. Don't judge yourself for how you feel.
- **Express yourself**: Find healthy ways to let your emotions out, such as:
    - Journaling
    - Talking with a trusted friend
    - Creating art or music
    - Engaging in physical activity
- **Practice self-compassion**: Be kind to yourself. You're doing the best you can in a difficult situation.
- **Seek support**: Don't hesitate to ask for help from family, friends, or professionals.
- **Plan for grief**: It's common to feel grief even before your loved one passes. Consider speaking with a counselor or joining a support group to help process your feelings.

Available Resources and Support Groups: You're Not Alone

There are many resources available to support you on this journey:

1. **Hospice-provided support**
    - Many hospice organizations offer counseling services for caregivers
    - Ask your hospice team about available resources

2. **Support groups**
    - In-person or online groups for caregivers
    - Grief support groups
    - Condition-specific support groups (e.g., for Alzheimer's or cancer caregivers)

3. **Online resources**
    - Caregiver.org
    - NationalHospiceFoundation.org
    - CancerCare.org (for cancer caregivers)

4. **Respite care**
    - Short-term care options to give you a break
    - Can be provided in-home or at a care facility

5. **Mental health professionals**
    - Therapists or counselors experienced in caregiver support
    - Your doctor can provide a referral if needed

6. **Religious or spiritual support**
    - Many faith communities offer support for caregivers
    - Chaplains can provide spiritual guidance and emotional support

Remember, seeking help is a sign of strength, not weakness. Don't hesitate to reach out and use the resources available to you.

Creating Your Support Network: Building Your Circle of Care

Consider making a list of people and resources you can turn to for different types of support. Here's a table to help you organize your support network:

Type of Support	Who to Contact	Contact Information
Emotional support	(e.g., close friend, counselor)	
Practical help	(e.g., neighbor, church member)	
Medical advice	(hospice nurse, primary care doctor)	
Spiritual guidance	(chaplain, religious leader)	

Fill in this table with the names and contact information of people you can contact when you need support. Keep it somewhere easily accessible.

Final Thoughts

Remember, by caring for your emotional needs and seeking support, you'll be better equipped to provide compassionate care for your loved one. You're doing meaningful work, and your well-being matters as much as the person you care for.

It's okay to have moments of doubt, exhaustion, or sadness. These feelings don't make you a lousy caregiver—they make you human. Be gentle with yourself, reach out for help when needed, and remember you're not alone.

Your love and care profoundly affect your loved one's life. Take pride in your comfort and support; don't forget to extend some of that care to yourself, too.

Legal and Ethical Considerations in Hospice Care: Honoring Your Loved One's Wishes

Understanding hospice care's legal and ethical aspects is essential when caring for a loved one. This knowledge can help you make informed decisions and ensure your loved one's wishes are respected. Let's explore these topics together.

Understanding Advanced Directives: Planning for Future Care

Advanced directives are legal documents that outline a person's wishes for end-of-life care. They're crucial for ensuring your loved one's preferences are followed, even if they can't communicate later.

Types of Advanced Directives:

1. **Living Will**: This document specifies the types of medical treatments a person does or doesn't want in specific situations.

2. **Healthcare Power of Attorney**: This appoints someone to make medical decisions on the patient's behalf if the patient is unable to do so.

3. **Do Not Resuscitate (DNR) Order**: This instructs healthcare providers not to perform CPR if the patient's heart or breathing stops.

Key Points About Advanced Directives:

- They should be created while the person is still able to make decisions
- They can be changed or revoked at any time by the person who created them
- Copies should be given to healthcare providers, family members, and the appointed healthcare power of attorney

Creating advanced directives can bring peace of mind to your loved one and your family. It ensures that care aligns with your loved one's values and wishes.

Power of Attorney Responsibilities: Advocating for Your Loved One

A power of attorney (POA) is a legal document that gives someone the authority to act on behalf of another person. In hospice care, this often refers to healthcare decisions.

Responsibilities of a Healthcare Power of Attorney:

- Making medical decisions when the patient can't
- Ensuring the patient's wishes, as outlined in their advanced directives, are followed
- Communicating with healthcare providers about treatment options
- Advocating for the patient's best interests

Essential Considerations for POAs:

1. Understand the patient's wishes thoroughly
2. Be prepared to make difficult decisions
3. Communicate openly with family members
4. Seek guidance from healthcare professionals when needed
5. Take care of your emotional well-being

Remember, having a power of attorney is a significant responsibility. It's okay to ask for help or support when you need it.

Making Informed Decisions About Comfort Care: Focusing on Quality of Life

Comfort care focuses on improving quality of life and managing symptoms rather than curing the underlying condition. Making decisions about comfort care can be challenging, but understanding the options can help.

Key Aspects of Comfort Care:

- Pain management
- Symptom control (e.g., nausea, shortness of breath)
- Emotional and spiritual support
- Respect for the patient's wishes

Steps for Making Informed Decisions:

1. **Gather Information**:
    - Ask the hospice team to explain all available options
    - Understand the benefits and potential side effects of each option

2. **Consider the Patient's Wishes**:
    - Refer to advanced directives
    - If possible, discuss options directly with the patient

3. **Weigh Quality of Life**:
    - Consider how each option might affect the patient's comfort and dignity

4. **Consult with Family**:
    - Discuss options with other family members
    - Aim for consensus, but remember that the patient's wishes come first

5. **Seek Guidance**:

- Don't hesitate to ask the hospice team for their professional opinion
- Consider speaking with a counselor or spiritual advisor if struggling with decisions

Important Reminders:

- There's often no single "right" answer
- Decisions can be revisited as circumstances change
- The goal is to honor the patient's wishes and ensure their comfort

Making decisions about end-of-life care is never easy, but you're not alone. Your hospice team is there to provide information, support, and guidance throughout this process. Don't hesitate to ask questions or express concerns.

Final Thoughts

By understanding advanced directives, power of attorney responsibilities, and the principles of comfort care, you can make informed decisions that respect your loved one's wishes and ensure their comfort and dignity.

Remember, your dedication to understanding these aspects of care is a profound expression of love and respect for your loved one. Sometimes, feeling overwhelmed or unsure is okay – these are complex issues, and you're doing your best to navigate them with compassion and care.

Take pride in honoring your loved one's wishes and providing the best care. Your love and attention to these critical details can bring comfort and peace to your loved one and your family during this challenging time.

The Dying Process at the End of Life

The following is from the author's book, Whispers of Time: Understanding the End-of-Life Timeline.

Living is a continuum. Scientifically, life begins at conception and progresses through various stages—from birth to childhood, adolescence, and adulthood. Throughout these stages, we live actively, often without considering the quality of life. As we approach the end of life, we enter a transitioning phase before actively dying.

This chapter will explore the dying process at the end of life, addressing common questions such as, "What is transitioning?" "How do I know if my loved one is actively dying?" and "What are the phases of dying?" The dying process can be divided into two main phases: transitioning and actively dying.

The Transitioning Phase

This phase marks the beginning of the dying process and can be confusing for loved ones. During this time, the person may still be eating, talking, or even somewhat mobile. This phase can last from a few seconds in sudden events like a heart attack to several weeks.

Signs that your loved one is transitioning include:

- Increased restlessness, which may indicate terminal restlessness.
- Subtle changes in complexion, becoming more pronounced as they near active dying. This may appear as pallor, greyness, or flushing.
- Reports of seeing and speaking to deceased loved ones.
- Spending more time alone, napping, or sleeping.
- Significant reduction in food intake over days or weeks.
- Noticeable changes in breathing patterns—faster, slower, or irregular.
- Periods of fixed staring, where they seem to look through you rather than at you.
- Loss of mobility and difficulty repositioning themselves.
- Trouble eating due to a weakening gag reflex.

As your loved one spends more time sleeping and showing these changes, they are likely nearing the end of the transitioning phase and moving into the actively dying stage.

The Actively Dying Phase

The active dying phase begins when your loved one becomes unconscious. Even experienced healthcare professionals may find it challenging to pinpoint the exact transition from the transitioning phase to active dying. Some professionals simplify this by informing families that their loved one is dying, thus combining the two phases.

Key characteristics of the actively dying phase include:

- They may be in a comatose-like state, often passing away in their sleep.
- The gag reflex is absent, so avoid giving food or drink to prevent choking.
- More noticeable changes in complexion.
- Respirations become a critical indicator, with patterns that may be extremely fast, slow, or fluctuating.
- Heart rate may become very fast or irregular.
- Ears may pin back, and earlobes may appear close to the neck.
- Development of a terminal fever that is resistant to medication.
- The presence of death gurgles due to accumulated secretions in the airway. This is not painful for them and can be managed by elevating the head of the bed and using prescribed medications.
- Possible mottling of the extremities due to circulatory changes.
- Unpreventable pressure injuries on bony areas like elbows, hips, knees, and tailbone.
- A significant amount of urine or a bowel movement may occur as the body prepares for the end.

In the final moments, their breathing will become more erratic. Secretions may emerge from their mouth, and they will take their last breath, which may sound like a gasp. This marks the end of their journey.

The Last Hours

Losing a loved one is profoundly difficult and sorrowful. You may wonder how much time they have left and how you can help them. You might also want to say goodbye and express your love. Some signs indicate your loved one is in their final hours, which can help you prepare.

Breathing Changes

In the last 24 to 36 hours, breathing patterns may change. They may breathe faster or slower, deeper or shallower, or stop and start. This is due to the weakening of their body and lungs. Gurgling or rattling sounds may occur because of excess saliva or mucus. You can help by raising your head, wiping your mouth, or offering ice chips.

Rapid Breathing

If breathing becomes very fast, with less than three minutes between breaths, the patient may have less than 12 hours left. Their heart may be beating fast, and their blood pressure may drop. Cold or blue hands and feet indicate poor blood circulation. They may be unable to talk or move due to a lack of oxygen to the brain. Comfort them by holding their hand, speaking softly, or playing soothing music.

Last Breath

They may cough or expel saliva or mucus when they take their last breath. This is normal and not painful. Reflex breaths may occur after the heart stops as the body shuts down. Check their pulse or listen to their chest to confirm they have passed. Then, say your goodbyes and thank them for being part of your life.

Understanding these phases and signs can help you navigate this challenging time with compassion and preparedness.

Conclusion

As we come to the end of this book, I hope you feel more equipped and supported in your role as a caregiver. Your journey is one of profound love and courage, and I want to take a moment to acknowledge your incredible work. Caring for a loved one in hospice is not easy, but it's one of the most meaningful gifts you can give.

Remember, it's okay to feel overwhelmed at times. It's normal to have questions, to feel uncertain, or to need help. These feelings don't make you a less capable caregiver - they make you human. Your walking path is challenging, and being gentle with yourself is essential.

Throughout this book, we've covered a lot of ground. You've learned about comfort medications - what they are, how they work, and when they might be used. This knowledge can help you feel more confident about your loved one's comfort. Remember, your hospice team is always there to answer questions or address concerns about these medications.

We've also explored caregiving techniques and ways to communicate effectively with your hospice team. These skills can help you navigate the day-to-day challenges of hospice care and ensure that your loved one's needs are met. Don't hesitate to contact your team for guidance or support - they're there for that.

You've delved into the legal and ethical aspects of end-of-life care. While these topics can be challenging, understanding them can help you honor your loved one's wishes and make informed decisions. Remember, you don't have to navigate these complex issues alone. Your hospice team, legal advisors, and support groups can all offer guidance.

Importantly, we've talked about taking care of yourself. While caring for others, it's easy to neglect our own needs. But your well-being matters, too. Taking time for self-care isn't selfish - it's necessary. It allows you to recharge and continue providing the best care possible for your loved one.

Beyond all this information, I hope you've felt a sense of companionship and understanding through these pages. Caring for someone at the end of life can sometimes feel isolating, but you're not alone in this experience. Millions of people have walked this path before you, and many are walking it alongside you.

Your dedication to your loved one is a beautiful gift. Try to find moments of connection, peace, and joy amid the challenges. These moments, however small, are precious. They're the threads that weave together the tapestry of your relationship, creating memories you'll always carry with you.

As you move forward, remember that you have support. Your hospice team, your personal support network, and the resources listed in this book are all here to help you. Don't hesitate to reach out when you need support, whether for practical help, emotional support, or just a listening ear.

Thank you for allowing me to be a part of your journey. Your compassion, care, and presence make a world of difference to your loved one. Even on the most challenging days, when you might not feel like you're doing enough, know that your efforts matter immensely.

Take pride in your comfort and support, but don't forget to extend some of that care to yourself. You're doing important and meaningful work, and it's okay to acknowledge that it can be challenging. Be kind to yourself, celebrate the small victories, and know you're making a difference daily.

As we close this book, I want to remind you of your strength. You're navigating one of life's most challenging journeys with love and dedication. Keep going, one day at a time, with love in your heart and hope by your side. Your loved one is fortunate to have you, and the care you're providing is a testament to the depth of your love.

Remember, this isn't goodbye. The resources in this book will always be here for you to refer back to, and your hospice team is just a phone call away. You've got this, and you're not alone. Wishing you moments of peace, strength, and connection as you continue on this journey of love and care.

Resources

National End-of-Life Doula Alliance (NEDA) at https://www.nedalliance.org/. NEDA provides resources, certification, and a directory of end-of-life doulas across the United States. This registry can help you find a certified doula to assist with end-of-life care, ensuring compassionate and professional support during this critical time.

International End-of-Life Doula Association (INELDA) at https://inelda.org/find-a-doula/ is another end-of-life doula organization if you are trying to find someone local to you.

Jamie Haberman, an RN with extensive hospice experience, runs Hospice Buddy at https://hospicebuddy.com/, where she offers daily coaching, support, and education for clients and caregivers, including 24/7 on-call availability. Because of her extensive hospice experience, she can often be a bridge between family members, caregivers, and the local hospice provider. She is a compassionate and excellent alternative if you are not in a position to hire an onsite end-of-life doula. The author of this book has no financial ties to Jamie Haberman or her business but does appreciate the care she continues to provide over the years.

Understanding Hospice Comfort Medications at https://compassioncrossing.info/understanding-hospice-comfort-medications/ -provides a condensed (compared to this book) summary of common hospice comfort medications.

Understanding PRN Medications for Comfort Care at https://compassioncrossing.info/understanding-prn-medications-for-comfort-care/ - provides a summary review of what PRN (as needed) means concerning hospice comfort care medications, including a review of maximum daily doses.

Understanding Discomfort: Distinguishing it from Pain While Caring for Your Terminally Ill Loved One at https://compassioncrossing.info/understanding-discomfort-distinguishing-it-from-pain-while-caring-for-your-terminally-ill-loved-one/ -- goes over the common myth that if one is not in pain, but uncomfortable then pain medication is not necessary.

[Morphine and Lorazepam are not euthanizing agents](https://compassioncrossing.info/morphine-and-lorazepam-are-not-euthanizing-agents/) at https://compassioncrossing.info/morphine-and-lorazepam-are-not-euthanizing-agents/, and [Common Misconceptions about Morphine and End-of-Life Medications](https://compassioncrossing.info/myths-about-morphine-used-at-the-end-of-life/) at https://compassioncrossing.info/myths-about-morphine-used-at-the-end-of-life/ go over the common misconceptions and myths about morphine concentrate, lorazepam, and the common end-of-life medications.

[Uncommon Opioid Side Effects to Know: How They Affect You and Your Family](https://compassioncrossing.info/uncommon-opioid-side-effects-to-know-how-they-affect-you-and-your-family/) at https://compassioncrossing.info/uncommon-opioid-side-effects-to-know-how-they-affect-you-and-your-family/ reviews the very uncommon side effects of morphine and other opioids and how to prevent or minimize the side effects.

[Recognizing and Treating Common End of Life Symptoms](https://compassioncrossing.info/guide-to-recognize-and-treat-common-end-of-life-symptoms/) at https://compassioncrossing.info/guide-to-recognize-and-treat-common-end-of-life-symptoms/ and [Crisis Management at End-of-Life](https://compassioncrossing.info/crisis-management-at-end-of-life/) at https://compassioncrossing.info/crisis-management-at-end-of-life/ reviews the crises that can occur at the end of life and the pharmacological and nonpharmacological means of dealing with them.

[CompassionCrossing.info](https://compassioncrossing.info/) at https://compassioncrossing.info/ is a free resource site with hundreds of articles covering various end-of-life topics, from specifics about diseases and disease processes to getting financial assistance to caregiver burnout and grief.

Author Bio

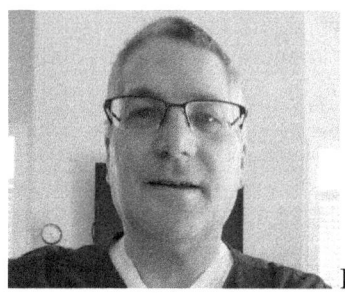 Peter Abraham, BSN, RN is an experienced nurse dedicated to supporting nurses, caregivers, families, and patients in their learning, growth, and well-being journey. Peter's nursing path encompasses practical experience as a cardiac telemetry nurse in a bustling cardiology unit at a Magnet-awarded teaching hospital. Additionally, Peter has fulfilled the role of a second-shift RN supervisor, overseeing an entire building in an SNF/LTC (Skilled Nursing Facility/Long-Term Care) setting with 151 residents. Remarkably, during the initial wave of COVID-19, the facility achieved an impressive close-to-100% recovery rate before operation warp speed was complete.

Furthermore, Peter's nursing career extends to rural home hospice care. As a visiting hospice registered nurse case manager, he offers compassionate care to patients in various settings, including private homes, personal care homes, assisted living facilities, skilled nursing facilities, and hospitals.

Moreover, Peter's desire to help others extends beyond his physical presence. At CompassionCrossing.Info, he writes articles to empower caregivers, family members, and fellow nurses in end-of-life care. Peter's drive to help others, which flows from his love of Christ Jesus, is a source of support and encouragement for all he reaches.

Other books by Peter Abraham include the following:

Empowering Excellence in Hospice: A Nurse's Toolkit for Best Practices series:

> Compliance-based, Eligibility Driven Hospice Documentation: Tips for Hospice Nurses
> Whispers of Time: Understanding the End-of-Life Timeline
> Terminal Clarity: Hospice Eligibility Guide for Nurses
> Mastering Recertifications: A Comprehensive Guide for Nurses

Compassionate Caregiving series:

> Daily Hospice Care Planner: Organize, Communicate, and Provide Consistent Care
> Dignity in Dying: A Thoughtful Approach to Voluntary Stopping Eating and Drinking
> Palliative Sedation: A Compassionate Approach
> Hospice Medication Handbook: A Caregiver's Guide to Comfort Medications
> Nourishing Hope: A Caregiver's Guide to End-of-Life Nutrition
> Validation and Compassion: A Guide to Connecting with Terminally Ill Loved Ones

Dementia Caregivers Essentials series:

> Dementia Caregiver Essentials (all ten books below in one)
>
> Anger Management in Dementia
> CPAP and Oxygen for Dementia
> Diabetes Care for Dementia
> Hallucination Management for Dementia
> Infection Awareness in Dementia
> Medication Compliance for Dementia
> Music Therapy for Dementia
> Nutrition for Dementia
> Placement for Dementia
> Sundowning Management for Dementia

Holistic Nurse: Skills for Excellence series

>Dementia Staging Mastery: A Nurse's Guide to Dementia Assessment

The above books can be found on Amazon at https://amzn.to/3YFBYQ0

Connect with Peter On:

Website: https://compassioncrossing.info/

www.ingramcontent.com/pod-product-compliance
Lightning Source LLC
Chambersburg PA
CBHW070406230526
45471CB00006B/2687